VEGETARIAN DIET RECIPES FOR BEGINNERS

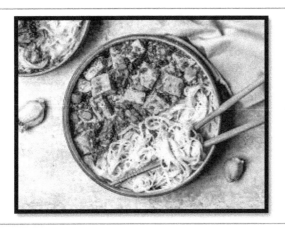

The Ultimate Beginner's Guide with More than 50 Vegetarian Meal Prep. Learn How to Prepare Delicious Dishes Quick and Easy, and Build a Complete and Healthy Meal Plan Made With the Best Flavors of the World and Mainly of the Mediterranean Diet. This Cookbook Is Suitable for All the Family

Isabel Lauren

Welcome

"VEGETARIAN DIET RECIPES FOR BEGINNERS"
is a cookbook I've realized after collecting the best vegetarian recipes I tasted in my travels around the world.

I personally love this type of dishes because I find them very healthy and free of contraindications, a tasty way to add more nutrients to our diet.

The benefits of vegetarian diet are so many, I want to remind you the most important below.

5 Most Benefits of Eating Vegetarian Dishes

1. MANAGE YOUR WEIGHT

Studies show that daily calories intake tends to be lower for people who eat vegetables. For instance, one observational study showed that people who regularly follow vegetarian diet had lower body weight and waist circumference than people who didn't. This is true in particular for starters.

2. BETTER DIET QUALITY

It is characterized by reduced fat and increased protein and fiber intakes. Most vegetarian dishes are, in fact, high in fiber. Fiber is known to increase feelings of fullness by delaying gastric emptying (the speed at which your stomach empties after eating) and increasing stomach volume by absorbing water – of which vegetables are rich - and swelling once it enters the stomach.

4

3. LONGEVITY THANKS TO LESS ANTIBIOTICS AND HORMONE

We know that in intensive farming, animals are often stuffed with hormones and antibiotics. And when we eat meat, they enters our organism, causing diseases, even as serious as cancer, over time. Eating vegetarian dishes helps you keep a regular and healthy diet, favoring longevity, as it drives away many diseases. And, of couse, this type of diet is on the side of the animals, and he fights intensive farming.

4. STAY HYDRATED

Water is essential for our health, and our total water intake may come from drinking water, water in beverages, or water in food (as is the case for salads and vegetables). If salads is not our thing during sport, it could be worth trying pre- or post-exercise to stay hydrated and with the right vitamins' amount included.

5. <u>PROTECT YOUR HEART AND BONES</u>

For healthy bone growth, a recommended full daily serving of vitamin K can be found in just 1 cup of watercress, radicchio or spinach. Or, for instance, Romaine lettuce contains two key nutrients in significant levels that help to protect the heart muscle. Finally, vegetarian diet is also good for the other organs, for the eyes, the skin, the muscles, and so on.

So, what are you waiting for?

Immediately start testing some recipes from the cookbook!
Good fun and if you want, add your personal pinch to my recipes!

Table of Content

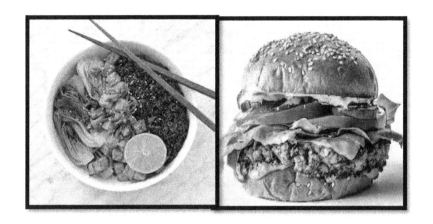

VEGETARIAN DIET RECIPES FOR BEGINNERS

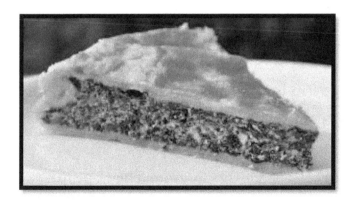

Vegetarian Spaghetti Sauce

Serves 8

Ingredients:

- 4 carrots, finely chopped
- 1 onion, finely chopped
- 1 tablespoon olive oil
- 2 garlic cloves, finely minced
- 14 oz canned cooked kidney beans, drained
- 14 oz canned cooked cannellini beans, drained
- 1 tablespoon chopped fresh basil
- 1 tablespoon chopped fresh oregano
- 2 x 14 oz cans chopped plum tomatoes
- 2 fl oz tomato purée
- 4 oz mushrooms, sliced
- 10 oz broccoli
- 1/4 teaspoon freshly ground black pepper

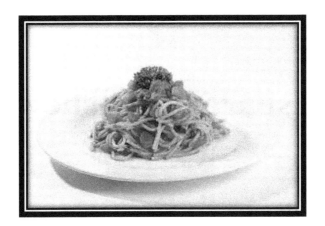

Procedure:

1. Sweat the carrots and onion in the oil in a large non-stick saucepan for 5 minutes until softened.
2. Add the garlic and sweat for a further 30 seconds.
3. Add the kidney and cannellini beans, basil, oregano, tomatoes, tomato purée and mushrooms.
4. Simmer, covered, for 25 minutes.
5. Add the broccoli and pepper, and cook for about 5 minutes until the broccoli is tender but still with a bite.
6. Serve hot over freshly cooked spaghetti.

Asparagus Cashew Stir-Fry

<u>Serves 4</u>

Ingredients:

- 8 oz raw cashew nuts
- 2 tablespoons sunflower oil
- 1 lb fresh asparagus
- 4 spring onions, chopped
- 1 red pepper, seeded and chopped
- 1 garlic clove, minced
- 2 lb freshly cooked brown rice, to serve

For the sauce

- 3 tablespoons light soy sauce
- 2 tablespoons cornflour
- 12 fl oz water
- 1 tablespoon minced fresh root ginger

14

- 1 teaspoon sesame oil

- 1/4 teaspoon crushed red pepper flakes

Procedure:

1. Spread the cashew nuts over a baking sheet.
2. Toast under a hot grill until golden, turning them frequently. Set aside.
3. To make the sauce, combine the soy sauce and cornflour in a small bowl, stirring until smooth.
4. Stir in the remaining sauce ingredients, and set aside.
5. Heat the oil in a wok over a medium-high heat.
6. Stir-fry the asparagus, spring onions, pepper and garlic until the vegetables are tender.
7. Stir the sauce mixture, pour it over the vegetables and stir-fry until the sauce is thickened and glossy
8. Reduce the heat and fold in the cashew nuts.
9. Cover and cook for 1 minute until the cashews are heated through.
10. Serve immediately with the hot brown rice.

Batter-Dipped Tofu

Serves 4–6

Ingredients:

- 8 oz firm tofu
- 4,5 oz plain flour
- 2 tablespoons toasted wheatgerm
- 1/2 teaspoon dried thyme
- 1/4 teaspoon dried dill
- 1/4 teaspoon garlic powder
- 1/4 teaspoon paprika

For the ginger dipping sauce

- 3,5 fl oz rice vinegar
- 2 oz granulated sugar
- 2 tablespoons light soy sauce
- 1 teaspoon cornflour
- 1 tablespoon finely minced fresh root ginger

- 1/4 teaspoon freshly ground black pepper
- 1 egg
- 1 tablespoon milk
- 1 teaspoon hot pepper sauce
- 2 tablespoons sunflower oil

Procedure:

1. To make the ginger dipping sauce, put the vinegar, sugar, soy sauce and 6 fl oz water in a small saucepan.

2. Bring to the boil, reduce the heat and simmer, stirring occasionally, for 5 minutes.

3. Meanwhile, in a small bowl, combine the cornflour and 1 teaspoon water, and stir into the sauce. Keep stirring until the sauce is clear and thickened.

4. Remove the pan from the heat, and stir in the ginger. Keep warm until needed.

5. Cut the tofu into 1 in squares about 8mm/14in thick. Set aside.

6. Combine the flour, wheatgerm, thyme, dill, garlic powder, paprika and pepper in a medium bowl.

7. In a separate bowl, lightly whisk the egg using a fork.

8. Add the milk and hot pepper sauce, and whisk again to combine.

9. Heat the oil in a large wok over a medium-high heat.

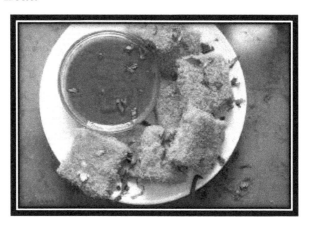

10. Piece by piece, dip the tofu in the flour, then in the egg mixture, and again in the flour.

11. Fry the pieces of tofu for about 3 minutes on each side until golden brown (if necessary, cook in batches so that the temperature of the oil does not drop). Drain on kitchen paper.

12. Serve immediately with a bowl of the ginger sauce for dipping.

Potato & Onion Pizza

Ingredients:

For the dough

- 1 teaspoon dried yeast
- 1/2 teaspoon granulated sugar
- pinch of salt
- 9 fl oz warm water
- 6 oz white bread flour
- 5 oz wholemeal plain flour

For the topping

- 1 red pepper
- 1 potato, very thinly sliced
- 1 large onion, sliced

- 4 oz soft goat's cheese, crumbled into small pieces
- 3 tablespoons capers, rinsed and drained
- 1 tablespoon dried oregano
- 1–2 tablespoons olive oil

Procedure:

1. To make the dough, mix the yeast, sugar, salt and water in a bowl.
2. Leave in a warm place for 10 minutes or until foamy. Sift both flours into a bowl.
3. Make a well, add the yeast mixture and mix to a firm dough. Knead on a lightly floured surface for 5 minutes or until smooth.
4. Put in a lightly oiled bowl, cover with cling film and leave in a warm place for 1–1,5 hours until doubled in size.
5. Preheat the oven to 400°F. Brush a 12 in pizza tray with oil.
6. Punch down the dough and knead for 2 minutes.
7. Roll out to a 14 in round. Put the dough on the tray and fold the edge over to form a rim.

8. To make the topping, cut the pepper into large flat pieces and remove the seeds.

9. Put the pepper, skin side up, under a hot grill until blackened.

10. Cool, then peel away and discard the skin, and slice the flesh.

11. Arrange the potato over the base with the pepper, onion and half of the cheese.

12. Sprinkle with the capers and oregano, and drizzle with a little oil.

13. Brush the crust edge with a little more oil, and bake the pizza in the oven for 15–20 minutes.

14. Add the remaining cheese and bake until the crust is golden and crisp.

15. Serve hot.

Brinjal Curry

Ingredients:

- 11 oz aubergine, cut into 1 in cubes
- 3 fl oz vegetable oil
- a little salt
- 1 teaspoon mustard seeds
- 20 curry leaves
- 1 teaspoon skinned and split
- urad dal
- 5 oz onions, finely sliced
- 7 oz tomatoes
- 1 tablespoon tomato purée
- 1/2 teaspoon chilli powder
- 1/2 teaspoon ground coriander
- 1/2 teaspoon ground turmeric

Procedure:

1. Soak the aubergine in cold water for 10 minutes. Drain and pat dry with kitchen paper.
2. In a large frying pan, heat 4 tablespoons of the oil over a medium heat.
3. Add the aubergine and a little salt, and cook for 10 minutes or until the aubergine is brown and soft.

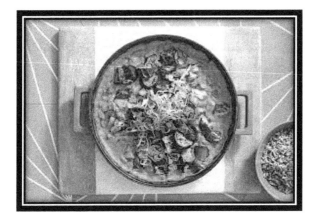

4. Drain the aubergine on kitchen paper, and set aside in a warm place.
5. Heat the remaining oil in the same pan. Add the mustard seeds and, as they begin to pop, add the curry leaves and urad dal.

6. Cook, stirring, for a few minutes or until the dal is golden, then add the onions and a little salt and cook until the onions are starting to colour, stirring occasionally.

7. Add the tomatoes, tomato purée, chilli powder, coriander and turmeric, and mix well.

8. Add the aubergine and cook for a further 5 minutes, stirring occasionally, until the tomatoes break down.

9. Transfer the mixture to a serving dish, and serve immediately.

Broccoli & Asparagus Fusilli

Ingredients:

- 8 oz dried fusilli
- 1 tablespoon olive oil
- 1 head broccoli, cut into florets
- 2 courgettes, sliced
- 8 oz fresh asparagus spears
- 4 oz mangetout
- 4oz frozen green peas
- 1 oz butter
- 2 tablespoons vegetable stock
- 4 tablespoons double cream
- 2 tablespoons chopped fresh flat-leaf parsley
- 2 tablespoons freshly grated Parmesan cheese

- salt
- freshly ground black pepper

Procedure:

1. Bring a large saucepan of lightly salted water to the boil. Add the fusilli and oil and cook until al dente.
2. Drain, return to the pan with a very little of the cooking liquid, cover and keep warm.
3. Meanwhile, steam the broccoli, courgettes, asparagus and mangetout over a pan of salted boiling water until they are just beginning to soften.
4. Remove from the heat and refresh in cold water. Drain and set aside.
5. Bring a small saucepan of lightly salted water to the boil. Add the peas and cook for 3 minutes, then drain.
6. Put the butter and stock in a saucepan over a medium heat.
7. When the butter has melted, add the vegetables, and toss until heated through.

8. Stir in the cream, and heat through gently without boiling. Season with salt and pepper.

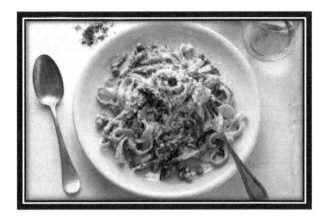

9. Transfer the pasta to a warmed serving dish, and stir in the parsley.
10. Spoon the sauce over the pasta, then sprinkle the Parmesan over the top.
11. Serve immediately.

Chickpea Chole

Serves 4–6

Ingredients:

- 3 tablespoons vegetable oil
- 1 onion, chopped
- 2 garlic cloves, crushed
- 1 in piece of fresh root ginger, grated
- 4 teaspoons ground cumin
- 1 tablespoon ground coriander
- 2 teaspoons chilli powder
- 14 oz canned chopped plum tomatoes
- 1,5 teaspoons Demerara sugar
- 2 tablespoons freshly squeezed lime juice
- 4 tablespoons torn fresh coriander leaves salt
- 1 teaspoon ground turmeric
- 2 x 14oz cans cooked chickpeas, drained and rinsed

Procedure:

1. Heat the oil in a heavy saucepan. Add the onion, garlic and ginger, and sweat over a gentle heat, stirring frequently, for about 5 minutes until softened.

2. Stir in the ground cumin, coriander, chilli powder and turmeric, and fry for 2 minutes until aromatic.

3. Add the chickpeas, tomatoes and sugar.

4. Season with salt, and stir to combine the ingredients.

5. Cover the pan and simmer the curry gently, stirring occasionally, for 10 minutes.

6. Stir in 1 tablespoon of the lime juice and the torn coriander leaves, and heat through for a further 2 minutes.

7. Taste the curry and add the remaining lime juice and more salt if necessary.

8. Serve hot.

Spinach & Mushroom Bhaji

Serves 8

Ingredients:

- 1 tablespoon mustard seeds
- 2 teaspoons coriander seeds
- 1 teaspoon cumin seeds
- 2 garlic cloves, roughly chopped
- 1 in piece of fresh root ginger, roughly chopped
- 2 fl oz vegetable oil
- 2 large onions, thinly sliced
- 2 teaspoons ground turmeric
- 1,5 teaspoons chilli powder
- 1 lb button mushrooms, thickly sliced
- 14 oz canned chopped plum tomatoes
- 2 lb fresh spinach, roughly shredded
- 4 tablespoons desiccated or shredded coconut, to garnish

- salt
- freshly ground black pepper

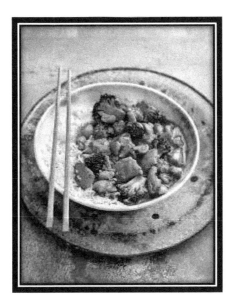

Procedure:

1. Put the mustard, coriander and cumin seeds in a large heavy flameproof casserole dish, and dry-roast over a medium heat for 2–3 minutes until aromatic, stirring all the time.
2. Remove from the dish and, using a mortar and pestle, crush into a paste with the garlic and ginger.

3. Heat the oil in the casserole dish, add the onions and sauté gently, stirring frequently, for about 10 minutes until soft and golden.
4. Add the spice paste, turmeric and chilli powder, and sauté gently, stirring all the time, for 5 minutes.
5. Add the mushrooms and stir to coat well with the spiced mixture, then add the tomatoes and bring to the boil, stirring all the time.
6. Simmer for 10 minutes, stirring occasionally.
7. Add the spinach and stir well, then season with salt and pepper.
8. Reduce the heat, cover and simmer for 15 minutes, stirring frequently to blend in the spinach.
9. Check the seasoning and adjust if necessary, then turn the mixture into a warmed serving dish.
10. Sprinkle with the coconut, and serve immediately.

Tofu With Mushrooms

Serves 4

Ingredients:

- 3 tablespoons light soy sauce
- 2 tablespoons Chinese rice wine
- 2 teaspoons brown sugar
- 1 garlic clove, crushed
- 1 tablespoon grated fresh root ginger
- 1/2 teaspoon five-spice powder
- 8 oz firm tofu, cut into 1 in cubes
- 6 dried Chinese mushrooms
- 1 teaspoon cornflour
- 2 tablespoons groundnut oil
- 6 spring onions, sliced into 1 in lengths, white and green parts separated

Procedure:

1. In a small bowl, mix together the soy sauce, rice wine, sugar, garlic, ginger and five-spice powder.
2. Put the tofu in a shallow dish.
3. Pour the marinade over, toss well and leave to marinate for about 30 minutes.
4. Drain, reserving the marinade.
5. Meanwhile, soak the dried Chinese mushrooms in warm water for 20–30 minutes until soft.
6. Drain, reserving 3 fl oz of the soaking liquid.
7. Squeeze out any excess liquid from the mushrooms, remove the stalks and slice the caps. In a bowl, blend the cornflour with the reserved marinade and mushroom soaking liquid.
8. Heat the oil in a wok or large heavy frying pan until hot. Add the tofu and stir-fry for 3 minutes or until evenly golden.
9. Remove from the wok using a slotted spoon, and set aside.
10. Add the mushrooms and white parts of the spring onions to the wok, and stir-fry for 2 minutes.

11. Pour in the marinade mixture and stir for 1 minute until thickened.

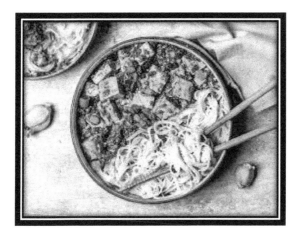

12. Return the tofu to the wok with the green parts of the spring onions. Simmer gently for 1–2 minutes.
13. Serve immediately with rice noodles.

Tofu & Broccoli Stir-Fry

<u>Serves 4</u>

Ingredients:

- 2 tablespoons dry sherry
- 2 tablespoons light soy sauce
- 4 teaspoons cornflour
- 1 teaspoon ground ginger
- 1 tablespoon vegetable oil
- 2 garlic cloves, minced
- 12 oz broccoli, cut into bite-size pieces
- 4 oz onion, cut into wedges
- 7 oz beansprouts
- 1 lb firm tofu, cut into 1/2 in pieces
- 9 oz freshly cooked brown rice, to serve

Procedure:

1. Put the sherry, soy sauce, cornflour and ginger in a bowl. Add 5 fl oz water, and stir together.
2. Heat the oil in a wok or large frying pan over a medium heat.
3. Add the garlic and stir-fry for 15 seconds.
4. Add the broccoli and onion, and stir-fry for 5 minutes, then add the beansprouts and stir-fry for a further 1 minute.
5. Tip the sauce mixture to the wok and stir until the sauce is thickened and glossy.
6. Stir in the tofu and heat through.
7. Serve with the hot brown rice.

Braised Chinese Vegetables

Serves 4

Ingredients:

- 1/2 oz dried Chinese mushrooms
- 8 oz firm tofu, cubed
- 2 fl oz vegetable oil
- 3 oz straw mushrooms
- 3 oz sliced bamboo shoots, drained
- 2 oz mangetout, topped and tailed
- 6 oz Chinese leaves such as pak choi, shredded
- 1 teaspoon salt
- 1/2 teaspoon soft brown sugar
- 1 tablespoon light soy sauce

Procedure:

1. Soak the Chinese mushrooms in cold water for 20–25 minutes, then drain, discarding any hard stalks.
2. Harden the tofu pieces by putting them in a wok of boiling water for about 2 minutes.Remove and drain.
3. Tip the water out of the wok, and wipe dry.
4. Heat the oil in the wok, and lightly brown the tofu pieces on both sides.
5. Remove with a slotted spoon and drain on kitchen paper.
6. Stir-fry the vegetables in the wok for 1,5 minutes, then add the tofu, salt, sugar and soy sauce.
7. Continue stirring for 1 minute, then cover and braise for 2–3 minutes.
8. Serve immediately.

Baked Peanut Tofu

Ingredients:

- 4 tablespoons smooth peanut butter
- 2 tablespoons tamari
- 1 garlic clove, crushed
- 1 lb firm tofu, cubed
- 1,5 tablespoons arrowroot

Procedure:

1. In a small bowl, mix together the peanut butter, tamari and garlic.
2. Slowly stir in 8 fl oz water. Mix well until the water in incorporated. Put the tofu in a shallow dish and pour the liquid over it.
3. Leave the tofu to marinate for at least 30 minutes.
4. Preheat the oven to 375°F.

5. Remove the tofu cubes from the marinade, and put them on a wellgreased baking tray.

6. Reserve the marinade to make the sauce.

7. Bake the tofu cubes in the oven for 30−45 minutes until the desired crispness is reached.

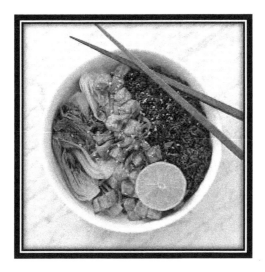

8. Mix the arrowroot with the remaining marinade.

9. Put the mixture in a heavy saucepan, and cook over a high heat, stirring constantly, until the sauce thickens.

10. Put the baked tofu on a bed of rice or pasta.

11. Cover with the sauce, and serve immediately

Cabbage & Tofu

<u>Serves 4</u>

Ingredients:

- 3 tablespoons vegetable oil
- 2,5 tablespoons tamari
- 1 tablespoon Worcestershire sauce
- 1/2 teaspoon ground allspice
- 1,2 lb firm tofu, cubed
- 1 onion, chopped
- 1,1 lb cabbage, shredded

For the sauce

- 2 tablespoons tomato purée
- 1 tablespoon vinegar
- 1 teaspoon dried dill
- 1 teaspoon salt
- 1/2 teaspoon paprika

Procedure:

1. Preheat the oven to 375°F.

2. In a baking dish, combine 1 tablespoon of the vegetable oil with the tamari, Worcestershire sauce and allspice to make a marinade.

3. Add the tofu and cook in the oven for about 35 minutes, turning the cubes two or three times during the cooking.

4. Sweat the onion in the remaining oil until translucent. Add the cabbage and cook, stirring occasionally, for 5 minutes.

5. Toss the cabbage mixture in the baked tofu.

6. Combine the sauce ingredients in a bowl.

7. Add 2 fl oz water, and pour the sauce over the cabbage, onion and tofu.

8. Stir to coat the ingredients evenly. Remove from the heat.

9. Cover and return the dish to the oven for 30 minutes.

10. Serve hot over rice or mashed potatoes.

Okra With Mango & Lentils

Serves 4

Ingredients:

- 4 oz green lentils such as Puy, picked and rinsed
- 2 fl oz corn oil
- 1/2 teaspoon onion seeds
- 2 onions, sliced
- 1 teaspoon fresh root ginger pulp
- 1 teaspoon garlic pulp
- 1,5 teaspoons chilli powder
- 1/4 teaspoon ground turmeric
- 1 teaspoon ground coriander
- 1 green or unripe mango, peeled and stoned
- 1 lb okra, chopped
- 2 fresh red chillies, seeded and sliced
- 1 tomato, sliced

Procedure:

1. Put the lentils a saucepan with just enough water to cover.
2. Bring to the boil, and boil for a couple of minutes, then reduce the heat.
3. immer for about 20 minutes until soft, topping up with water if necessary. Drain.
4. Heat the oil in a wok or large heavy frying pan.
5. Add the onion seeds and fry until they begin to pop.
6. Add the onions and sauté until they are golden.
7. Reduce the heat and add the ginger, garlic, chilli powder, turmeric and coriander. Stir for a minute or so.
8. Slice the mango, then add with the okra.
9. Stir well, then add the chillies. Stir-fry for about 3 minutes until the okra is well cooked.
10. Stir in the cooked lentils and tomato, then cook for a further 3 minutes.
11. Serve immediately.

Spicy Okra

Ingredients:

- 3 tablespoons ghee or butter
- 1 large onion, sliced
- 2 garlic cloves, sliced
- 1 tablespoon ground coriander
- 1 teaspoon freshly ground black pepper
- 1 teaspoon ground turmeric
- 1/2 teaspoon salt
- 1 lb okra, topped, tailed and cut into ½ in pieces
- 1/2 teaspoon garam masala

Procedure:

1. Melt the ghee or butter in a large frying pan over a low heat.
2. Add the onions and garlic, and sweat until soft but not caramelized.

3. Add the ground coriander, pepper, turmeric and salt, and sweat for a further 4 minutes, stirring constantly.
4. Add the okra.
5. Coat with the mixture, then stir in 1 pt water.
6. Cover and simmer for 5–10 minutes until the okra is tender.
7. Stir in the garam masala, and serve immediately.

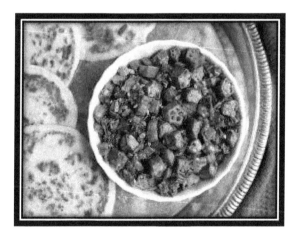

Chestnut & Sprout Sauté

Serves 8

Ingredients:

- 2 lb fresh chestnuts
- 1 pt vegetable stock
- 2 lb fresh Brussels sprouts
- 4 oz butter
- 1 lb onions, quartered, with layers separated
- 8 oz celery, trimmed and cut into 1 in pieces
- freshly grated zest of 1 lemon
- salt
- freshly ground black pepper

Procedure:

1. Snip the brown outer skins of the chestnuts, and put the chestnuts in boiling water for 3–5 minutes.

2. Lift out a few at a time, then peel off both the brown and inner skins.

3. Put the chestnuts in a saucepan, cover with the stock and simmer for 40–45 minutes until tender. Drain well.

4. Meanwhile, trim the sprouts and, with a sharp knife, make a cross in the stalk end of each one.

5. Cook the sprouts in boiling salted water for 3–4 minutes only; drain well.

6. Melt the butter in a large heavy frying pan.

7. Add the onions, celery and lemon zest, and sauté for 2–3 minutes until softened.

8. Add the cooked chestnuts and sprouts, and season with salt and pepper.

9. Sauté for a further 1–2 minutes, and serve immediately.

Vegetable Raisin Curry

Serves 4

Ingredients:

- 1 tablespoon vegetable oil
- 1 large onion, coarsely chopped
- 1 teaspoon freshly minced garlic
- 1 tablespoon plain flour
- 2 teaspoons curry powder
- 1/4 teaspoon cayenne pepper
- 1 lb frozen mixed vegetables
- 4 oz raisins
- 1/2 teaspoon salt
- 18 fl oz vegetable stock
- 8 oz quick-cooking couscous
- 2 oz sliced almonds, toasted

50

Procedure:

1. In a frying pan, heat the oil and sauté the onion and garlic for a few minutes until soft. Stir in the flour, curry powder and cayenne, and cook for 1 minute, stirring constantly.

2. Stir in the vegetables, raisins, salt and half of the stock.

3. Cover and bring to a boil over a high heat.

4. Reduce the heat to low and continue cooking, covered, for 10 minutes, stirring occasionally.

5. Bring the remaining stock to the boil in a small saucepan.

6. Stir in the couscous and remove from the heat.

7. Cover and leave to stand for 5 minutes or until the liquid is absorbed. Fluff the grains with a fork.

8. To serve, put the curry on a bed of couscous, sprinkle with the almonds and serve immediately.

Casseroled Beans & Penne

<u>Serves 4</u>

Ingredients:

- 8 oz dried haricot beans, soaked overnight, rinsed and drained
- 1,5 pt vegetable stock
- 3,5 fl oz olive oil
- 2 large onions, sliced
- 2 garlic cloves, chopped
- 2 bay leaves
- 1 teaspoon dried oregano
- 75ml/3fl oz red wine
- 2 tablespoons tomato purée
- 8 oz dried penne
- 2 celery sticks, sliced
- 4 oz mushrooms, sliced
- 8 oz tomatoes, sliced

- 1 teaspoon muscovado sugar
- 4 tablespoons dried white breadcrumbs
- salt
- freshly ground black pepper

Procedure:

1. Preheat the oven to 350°F.
2. Put the haricot beans in a large heavy saucepan, and add enough cold water to cover.
3. Bring to the boil and continue to boil vigorously for 20 minutes. Drain.
4. Put the beans in a large flameproof casserole dish.
5. Add the vegetable stock, and stir in all but 1 tablespoon of the oil, the onions, garlic, bay leaves, oregano, wine and tomato purée.
6. ring to the boil, then cover and cook in the oven for 2 hours.
7. Bring a large saucepan of lightly salted water to the boil. Add the penne and the remaining oil, and cook for about 3 minutes. Drain.

8. Add the penne, celery, mushrooms and tomatoes to the casserole dish, and season with salt and pepper.
9. Stir in the muscovado sugar, and sprinkle the breadcrumbs over the top.
10. Cover the dish and cook in the oven for a further 1 hour.
11. Serve hot.

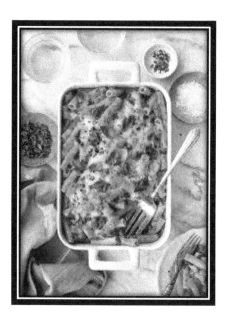

Courgette Quiche

Ingredients:

For the pastry

- 6 oz plain flour
- pinch of salt
- 4 oz butter, cut into pieces
- 4 oz Cheddar cheese, grated
- 1 egg yolk, beaten
- a little egg white, to seal

For the filling

- 12 oz courgettes, cut into 1 in chunks
- 3 eggs
- 5 fl oz double cream
- 2 teaspoons chopped fresh basil
- finely grated zest of 1 lime

- a little egg white
- salt
- freshly ground black pepper

Procedure:

1. Make the pastry by sifting the flour into a bowl with a pinch of salt.
2. Add the butter in pieces and rub in thoroughly with fingertips until the mixture resembles fine breadcrumbs.
3. Stir in the cheese, then the egg yolk. Gather the mixture together with your fingers to make a smooth ball of dough.
4. Wrap the dough in cling film and chill in the refrigerator for about 30 minutes.
5. Preheat the oven to 400°F.
6. To make the filling, plunge the courgette pieces into salted boiling water, bring back to the boil, then simmer for 3 minutes. Drain and set aside.

7. Put the eggs in a jug, and beat lightly together with the cream. Stir in the basil and lime zest, and sprinkle with salt and pepper. Set aside.

8. Roll out the chilled dough on a floured work surface, and use to line a loose-bottomed 9 in flan tin.

9. Refrigerate for 15 minutes.

10. Prick the base of the dough with a fork, then line with foil. Stand the tin on a preheated baking sheet, and bake in the oven for 10 minutes.

11. Remove the foil and brush the inside of the pastry case with the egg white to seal.

12. Return to the oven for 5 minutes.

13. Stand the courgette chunks upright in the pastry case, then slowly pour in the egg and cream mixture.

14. Return to the oven for 20 minutes until set and golden.

15. Serve hot or cold.

Pineapple & Coconut Curry

Serves 6

Ingredients:

- 2 tablespoons groundnut oil
- 1 red onion, sliced
- 2 garlic cloves, crushed
- 2 whole cloves, bruised
- 2 in cinnamon stick
- 1/4 teaspoon ground cardamom
- 1/2 teaspoon ground turmeric
- 2 teaspoons ground cumin
- 1 tablespoon ground coriander
- 1 large fresh red chilli, deseeded and sliced
- 1/2 teaspoon salt
- 1 ripe pineapple, peeled, cored and cut into 1 in chunks

- 3 oz creamed coconut, dissolved in 9 fl oz boiling water

Procedure:

1. Heat the oil in a flameproof casserole dish, add the onion, garlic, cloves and cinnamon stick, and sauté over a gentle heat, stirring frequently, for about 5 minutes until softened.

2. Add the ground cardamom, turmeric, cumin, coriander, chilli and salt to the pan, and sauté for a further 2 minutes. Add the pineapple chunks and stir well to coat them evenly in the spice mixture.

3. Stir in the coconut milk, stir to mix and bring to the boil. Reduce the heat and cook the curry very gently, stirring frequently, for 2–3 minutes until the pineapple is tender but not mushy and the sauce is very thick. Taste and adjust the seasoning if necessary, and serve immediately.

Potato Curry

Ingredients:

- 2 tablespoons vegetable oil
- 1 teaspoon mustard seeds
- 2 dried red chillies
- 3 curry leaves
- 2 onions, chopped
- 1/2 teaspoon ground coriander
- 1/2 teaspoon garam masala
- 1/2 teaspoon ground turmeric
- 1/4 teaspoon chilli powder
- 2 tomatoes, quartered
- 14 oz potatoes, cut into chunks
- 4 fl oz coconut milk

Procedure:

1. Heat the oil in a large saucepan over a medium heat.
2. Add the mustard seeds, chillies and curry leaves.
3. As the mustard seeds begin to pop, add the onions and sauté, stirring, until lightly browned.
4. Stir in the coriander, garam masala, turmeric and chilli powder. Sauté for a minute or so.
5. Add the tomatoes and cook for 5 minutes.
6. Add the potatoes and cook over a gentle heat for 5 minutes, stirring constantly.
7. Pour in the coconut milk and 125ml/4fl oz water.
8. Cook for 15–20 minutes until the potatoes are tender and serve hot.

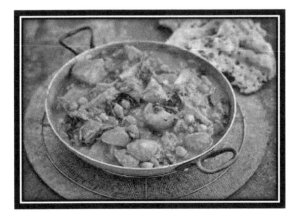

Mushroom Vol-Au-Vent

Serves 4

Ingredients:

- 1,1 lb ready-prepared puff pastry
- 1 egg, beaten, for glazing

For the filling

- 1 oz butter
- 1,5 lb mixed mushrooms
- 3,5fl oz white wine
- 4 tablespoons double cream
- 2 tablespoons chopped fresh chervil
- salt
- freshly ground black pepper

Procedure:

1. Preheat the oven to 425°F. Roll out the pastry to a 8 in square on a lightly floured work surface.
2. Using a sharp knife, mark a square 1 in from the pastry edge, cutting halfway through the pastry. Score the top in a diagonal pattern. Knock up the edges with a kitchen knife and put on a baking tray. Brush the top with beaten egg.
3. Bake in the oven for 35 minutes or until puffed and golden.
4. Cut out the central square. Discard the soft pastry inside the case, leaving the base intact. Return to the oven, with the central square, for 10 minutes.
5. Make the filling by melting the butter in a frying pan and sautéeing the mushrooms, stirring, over a high heat for 3 minutes.
6. Add the wine and cook, stirring occasionally, for 10 minutes, until the mushrooms have softened.
7. Stir in the cream and chervil, and season with salt and pepper.
8. Pile the filling into the pastry case. Top with the pastry square, and serve immediately.

Quinoa & Butter Beans

<u>Serves 4</u>

Ingredients:

- 1 oz butter
- 6 oz onion, finely chopped
- 1 tablespoon minced fresh ginger
- 6 fl oz freshly squeezed orange juice
- 2 tablespoons clear honey
- 1/2 teaspoon salt
- 1/4 teaspoon ground coriander
- 1/4 teaspoon ground cardamom
- 1/8 teaspoon ground nutmeg
- 8 oz sweet potato, cut into 1/2 in pieces
- 8 oz butternut squash, cut into 1/2 in pieces

- 8 oz canned cooked butter beans, drained and rinsed
- 8 oz quinoa
- 2 oz cranberries, chopped

Procedure:

1. Melt the butter in a large saucepan over a medium-high heat.
2. Add the onion and ginger, and sauté, stirring, until the onion is softened.
3. Stir in the orange juice, 5 fl oz water, honey, salt, coriander, cardamom and nutmeg, and bring to the boil.
4. Stir in the sweet potato and squash, and bring back to the boil.
5. Reduce the heat to a simmer and cook, uncovered, for 7 minutes.
6. Stir in the butter beans and quinoa, and return to the boil.
7. Reduce the heat and simmer, covered, for 15 minutes.
8. Stir in the cranberries and simmer, covered, for a further 5 minutes.

Chargrilled Peppers & Sweet Potatoes

Ingredients:

- 2 red peppers
- 2 yellow peppers
- 2 green peppers
- 1 sweet potato
- about 2 tablespoons olive oil

For the dressing

- 1 teaspoon cumin seeds
- 2 teaspoons clear honey
- 2 tablespoons balsamic vinegar
- 1 tablespoon walnut oil
- 1 tablespoon olive oil
- salt
- freshly ground black pepper

Procedure:

1. Halve the peppers lengthways and discard the stalks, cores and seeds. Cut each half lengthways into four pieces.
2. Peel the sweet potato and slice into rings about 1/4 in thick.
3. To make the dressing, in a small frying pan, dry-roast the cumin seeds over a low heat for a few minutes until aromatic, taking care not to burn them.
4. Put them in a bowl with the honey, vinegar and oils, and whisk together. Season with salt and pepper.
5. Heat a ridged cast-iron grill pan until very hot. Put the sweet potato slices on the pan, and lightly brush each piece with a little of the oil.
6. Cook for about 10 minutes, turning the pieces over once, then remove from the pan and keep warm.
7. Add half the pepper pieces, brush with a little oil and cook for about 8 minutes, turning them over several times.

8. Remove and add to the sweet potatoes, then repeat with the remaining peppers.

9. To serve, put the vegetables on a large shallow dish, and drizzle the dressing over them.

10. Serve warm with rice.

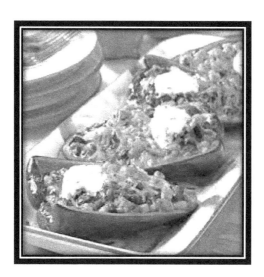

Couscous Vegetable Loaf

Ingredients:

- 2 pt vegetable stock
- 1 lb quick-cooking couscous
- 1 oz butter
- 8 large fresh basil leaves, chopped
- 2 oz fresh basil, chopped
- 5 oz sun-dried peppers in oil
- 3 tablespoons olive oil
- 2 garlic cloves, crushed
- 1 onion, finely chopped
- 1 tablespoon ground coriander
- 1 teaspoon ground cinnamon
- 1 teaspoon garam marsala

- 8 oz cherry tomatoes, quartered
- 1 courgette, finely chopped
- 5 oz canned sweetcorn

For the dressing

- 3 fl oz freshly squeezed orange juice
- 1 tablespoon freshly squeezed lemon juice
- 3 tablespoons chopped fresh flat-leaf parsley
- 1 teaspoon honey
- 1 teaspoon ground cumin kernels, drained

Procedure:

1. Bring the stock to the boil in a saucepan.
2. Put the couscous and butter in a large bowl, cover with the hot stock and set aside for 10 minutes.
3. Heat 1 tablespoon of the oil in a large frying pan, and sweat the garlic and onion over a low heat for 5 minutes or until the onion is soft.
4. Add the spices and cook for 1 minute until fragrant. Remove from the pan.

5. Add the remaining oil to the pan and sauté the tomatoes, courgette and corn over a high heat in batches until soft.

6. Line a 5 pt loaf tin with cling film, allowing it to overhang the sides. Arrange the basil leaves along the bottom of the tin.

7. Drain the peppers, reserving 2 tablespoons oil, then roughly chop.

8. Add the garlic and onion mixture, sautéed vegetables, pepper and chopped basil to the couscous and mix together.

9. Press the mixture into the tin, and fold the cling film over to cover. Weigh down and refrigerate overnight.

10. To make the dressing, put all the ingredients in a screwtop glass jar, and shake well to combine.

11. Turn out the loaf and serve with the dressing and potatoes.

Tabbouleh & Tofu

Ingredients:

- 8 oz bulgur wheat
- 1 pt lukewarm water
- 3 fl oz olive oil
- 3 fl oz freshly squeezed lemon juice
- 4 garlic cloves, finely chopped
- 1 oz chopped fresh flat-leaf parsley
- 1 oz chopped fresh mint
- 4 tomatoes, peeled and chopped
- 1 bunch of spring onions, trimmed and finely chopped
- 7 oz marinated tofu
- salt
- freshly ground black pepper

Procedure:

1. Soak the bulgur wheat in the water for 30 minutes, then drain in a sieve, squeezing it with your hands to extract the water.

2. Tip out onto a clean tea towel, gather the corners together and wring out the water so that the bulgur is as dry as possible.

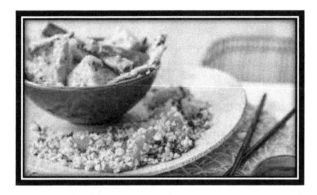

3. Whisk the oil and lemon juice together in a bowl with the garlic, parsley and mint. Season with salt and pepper.

4. Add the bulgur and toss to coat in the dressing.

5. Add the tomatoes, spring onions and tofu.

6. Fork through until evenly distributed. Taste and adjust the seasoning.

7. Serve at room temperature.

Pepper & Onion Pizza

Ingredients:

- 2 large red peppers
- 4 tablespoons olive oil, plus extra for drizzling
- 2 large onions, sliced
- 1 lb white bread and pizza mix
- 7 oz mozzarella cheese, sliced
- 14 oz canned chopped plum tomatoes, drained
- 3 garlic cloves, thinly sliced
- salt
- freshly ground black pepper

Procedure:

1. Preheat the oven to 400°F.

2. Halve the peppers and roast in the oven until blackened all over.

3. Leave until cold enough to handle, then carefully peel off the skins.

4. Cut the flesh into thick strips, discarding the seeds. Leave the oven on.

5. Heat 2 tablespoons olive oil in a frying pan, and sweat the onions gently for 5 minutes until softened but not coloured. Set aside.

6. Make up the pizza dough following the packet instructions, substituting 2 tablespoons oil for a similar amount of the liquid measurement.

7. Roll out into a 12 in round on a floured work surface, then slide onto a baking tray.

8. Cover the pizza base with the mozzarella.

9. Scatter over the tomatoes, onions and peppers, then the garlic.

10. Season with salt and pepper, drizzle with olive oil and leave in a warm place for 20–30 minutes until the dough has doubled in thickness.

11. Bake in the oven for 15–20 minutes until golden and bubbling.

Spicy Japanese Noodles

Serves 4

Ingredients:

- 1,1 lb fresh Japanese noodles such as soba
- 1 tablespoon sesame oil
- 1 tablespoon sesame seeds
- 1 tablespoon sunflower oil
- 1 red onion, sliced
- 4 oz mangetout
- 6 oz carrots, thinly sliced
- 12 oz white cabbage, shredded
- 3 tablespoons sweet chilli sauce
- 2 spring onions, sliced

Procedure:

1. Bring a large saucepan of water to the boil. Add the noodles to the pan, and cook for 2–3 minutes.
2. Drain the noodles thoroughly.
3. Toss the noodles with the sesame oil and sesame seeds, and set aside.
4. Heat the sunflower oil in a large preheated wok.
5. Add the onion slices, mangetout, carrot slices and shredded cabbage, and stir-fry for about 5 minutes.
6. Add the sweet chilli sauce to the wok and cook, stirring occasionally, for a further 2 minutes.
7. Add the sesame noodles to the wok, toss thoroughly to combine and heat for a further 2–3 minutes.
8. Transfer the Japanese noodles and spicy vegetables to warm individual serving bowls, scatter over the spring onions and serve immediately.

Pasticcio

Ingredients:

- 1 red pepper, seeded and chopped
- 1 yellow pepper, seeded and chopped
- 1 aubergine, chopped
- 1 large courgette, chopped
- 2 garlic cloves, crushed
- 1 teaspoon dried mixed herbs
- 2 tablespoons olive oil
- 8 oz short pasta such elbow macaroni
- 7 fl oz vegetable stock
- 11 oz mozzarella cheese, diced
- salt
- freshly ground black pepper

For the tomato sauce

- 1 oz sun-dried tomatoes, chopped
- 14 oz canned chopped tomatoes
- 1/2 teaspoon sugar
- 1,1 lb ripe plum tomatoes, seeded and chopped
- 2 teaspoons balsamic vinegar

Procedure:

1. Preheat the oven to 400°F.
2. For the tomato sauce, put the sun-dried tomatoes in a saucepan with the canned tomatoes and sugar.
3. Bring to a simmer, and continue to simmer for 5 minutes.
4. Add the diced plum tomatoes and cook gently for 10 minutes, stirring occasionally.
5. Remove the pan from the heat, and stir in the balsamic vinegar. Set aside.
6. Put the peppers, aubergine and courgette chunks in a large non-stick roasting tin, and mix in the garlic, dried herbs and oil.

7. Season with salt and pepper. Roast in the oven for 30–40 minutes, stirring occasionally.

8. Cook the pasta in salted boiling water until al dente. Drain well. In a separate pan, heat the

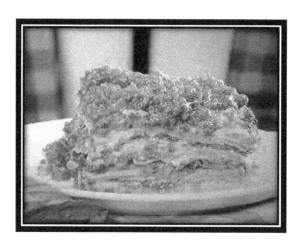

tomato sauce with the stock.

9. Put the vegetables and pasta in a large baking dish, and mix well. Pour the tomato sauce over them and mix through, then put the mozzarella cubes on top.

10. Bake in the oven for 15–20 minutes until melted and golden.

11. Leave to stand for 5–10 minutes before serving.

Vegetable biryani

Serves 4

Ingredients:

- 4 tablespoons vegetable oil
- 2 onions, sliced
- 2 garlic cloves, crushed
- 1 in piece of fresh root ginger, sliced
- 1 teaspoon ground turmeric
- 1/2 teaspoon chilli powder
- 1 teaspoon ground coriander
- 2 teaspoons ground cumin
- 4 oz red lentils, picked and rinsed
- 3 tomatoes, chopped
- 1 aubergine, cut into cubes
- 3 pt vegetable stock
- 1 red pepper, seeded and diced

- 12 oz basmati rice
- 4 oz French beans, halved
- 8 oz cauliflower florets
- 8 oz mushrooms, quartered
- 2 oz unsalted cashew nuts

Procedure:

1. Heat the oil in a saucepan, add the onions and fry gently for 2 minutes.
2. Stir in the garlic, ginger and spices, and fry gently, stirring frequently, for 1 minute.
3. Add the lentils, tomatoes, aubergine and 1 pt of the stock. Stir well, then cover and simmer gently for 20 minutes.
4. Add the pepper and cook for a further 10 minutes or until the lentils are tender and all the liquid has been absorbed.
5. Meanwhile, rinse the rice under cold running water. Drain and place in another pan with the remaining stock.

6. Bring to the boil, add the French beans, cauliflower and mushrooms, then cover and cook gently for 15 minutes or until the rice and vegetables are tender.

7. Remove from the heat and set aside, covered, for 10 minutes.

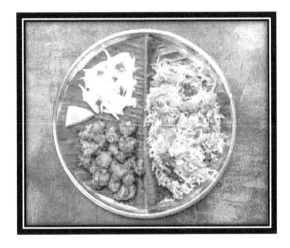

8. Add the lentil mixture and the cashews to the cooked rice, and mix lightly together.

9. Serve hot.

Stuffed Peppers

Ingredients:

- 3 green peppers
- 3 red peppers
- 2 yellow peppers
- 5 tablespoons olive oil
- 2 onions, chopped
- 4 garlic cloves, crushed
- 12 oz tomatoes, seeded and chopped
- 1 tablespoon tomato purée
- 1 teaspoon sugar
- 3 tablespoons chopped fresh coriander leaves
- 8 oz risotto rice such as Arborio or Carnaroli
- 1/2 teaspoon ground cinnamon
- salt
- freshly ground black pepper

Procedure:

1. Cut a slice off the top of each pepper and reserve. Remove the cores, seeds and membranes, and discard.

2. Wash the peppers and pat dry with kitchen paper.

3. Heat 4 tablespoons of the oil in a large frying pan, add the peppers and sauté gently for 10 minutes, turning them frequently so that they soften and colour on all sides.

4. Remove from the pan with a slotted spoon, and drain on kitchen paper.

5. To make the stuffing, drain off all but 2 tablespoons of oil from the pan, then add the onion and garlic, and seat very gently for about 15 minutes.

6. Add the tomatoes and sweat gently to soften, stirring constantly.

7. Increase the heat and cook rapidly to drive off the liquid – the mixture should be thick and pulpy.

8. Reduce the heat, and add the tomato purée, sugar.

9. Season with salt and pepper, and simmer gently for 5 minutes. Remove the pan from the heat and

stir in the chopped fresh coriander and the risotto rice.

10. Spoon the stuffing into the peppers, dividing it equally between them.

11. Stand the peppers close together in a flameproof casserole dish. Sprinkle with the cinnamon, then the remaining 1 tablespoon oil.

12. Put the reserved 'lids' on top.

13. Carefully pour 5 fl oz water into the bottom of the pan, then bring to the boil.

14. Reduce the heat, cover with a plate or saucer that just fits inside the rim of the dish, then place weights on top.

15. Simmer gently for 1 hour, then remove from the heat and leave to cool. Chill in the refrigerator overnight, with the weights still on top.

16. Serve the stuffed peppers chilled, with garlic bread and a salad.

Gado Gado

Ingredients:

- 4 oz white cabbage, shredded
- 4 oz French beans, each cut into three
- 4 oz carrots, cut into matchsticks
- 4 oz cauliflower florets
- 4 oz beansprouts

For the dressing

- 4 fl oz vegetable oil
- 4 oz unsalted peanuts
- 2 garlic cloves, crushed
- 1 small onion, finely chopped
- 1/2 teaspoon chilli powder
- 1/2 teaspoon soft brown sugar

- salt
- juice of 1/2 lemon

Procedure:

1. Cook the vegetables separately in a saucepan of salted boiling water for 4–5 minutes. Drain well and chill.
2. To make the dressing, heat the oil in a frying pan and fry the peanuts, tossing frequently, for 3–4 minutes.
3. Remove from the pan with a slotted spoon, and drain on kitchen paper.
4. Chop the peanuts in a blender or food processor, or crush with a rolling pin, until fine but not ground to a powder – leave a little texture.
5. Pour all but 1 tablespoon of the oil from the pan, and fry the garlic and onion for 1 minute.
6. Add the chilli powder, sugar, a pinch of salt and 3/4 pt water, and bring to the boil.
7. Stir in the peanuts, reduce the heat and simmer for 4–5 minutes until the sauce thickens.

8. Add the lemon juice and set aside to cool.

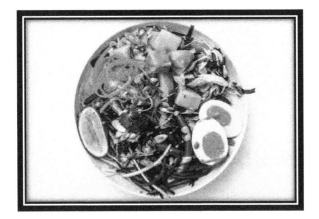

9. Arrange the cold vegetables in a serving dish, and put the peanut dressing in a small bowl in the centre.

10. Serve.

Nut Roast

Ingredients:

- 2 tablespoons olive oil
- 1 large onion, diced
- 2 garlic cloves, crushed
- 10 oz mushroom caps, wiped with damp kitchen paper and finely chopped
- 7 oz raw cashew nuts
- 7 oz Brazil nuts
- 4 oz Cheddar cheese, grated
- 1 oz Parmesan cheese, freshly grated
- 1 egg, lightly beaten
- 2 tablespoons chopped fresh chives
- 3 oz fresh wholemeal breadcrumbs
- salt
- freshly ground black pepper

Procedure:

1. Grease a 5,5 x 8,5 in loaf tin, and line the bottom with baking parchment.
2. Heat the oil in a frying pan over a medium heat, and add the onion, garlic and mushrooms.
3. Sweat until soft, then cool.
4. Process the nuts in a blender or food processor until finely chopped.
5. Preheat the oven to 180°C/350°F/Gas mark 4.
6. Combine the cooled mushrooms, chopped nuts, Cheddar, Parmesan, egg, chives and breadcrumbs in a bowl.
7. Mix well and season with salt and pepper.
8. Press the mixture into the loaf tin, and bake for 45 minutes or until firm.
9. Remove from the oven and leave in the tin for 5 minutes, then turn out and cut into slices.
10. Serve hot with potatoes.

Tomatoes Au Gratin

Serves 6

Ingredients:

- 2 lb tomatoes
- 2 oz butter, softened
- 3 garlic cloves, chopped
- 1 teaspoon sugar
- 4 teaspoons chopped fresh basil
- 10 fl oz double cream
- 2 oz dried breadcrumbs
- 1 oz Parmesan cheese, freshly grated
- salt
- freshly ground black pepper

Procedure:

1. Preheat the oven to 350°F.

2. Put the tomatoes in a bowl of just-boiled water, and leave for 30 seconds.

3. Peel off the skin and thinly slice the flesh.

4. Brush the inside of an ovenproof dish liberally with some of the butter.

5. Arrange a layer of tomato slices in the bottom of the dish, then sprinkle with a little of the garlic, sugar and basil.

6. Season with salt and pepper. Pour over a thin layer of cream.

7. Repeat these layers until all the ingredients have been used.

8. Mix the breadcrumbs and Parmesan together, then sprinkle over the top of the tomatoes and cream. Dot with the remaining butter.

9. Bake in the oven for 20–30 minutes until the topping is golden brown.

10. Serve hot.

Spinach & Ricotta Pie

<u>Serves 4</u>

Ingredients:

- 8 oz spinach
- 1 oz pine nuts
- 4 oz ricotta cheese
- 2 large eggs, beaten
- 2 oz ground almonds
- 1,5 oz Parmesan cheese, freshly grated
- 9 oz ready-prepared puff pastry
- 1 small egg, beaten, to glaze

Procedure:

1. Preheat the oven to 425°F.

2. Rinse the spinach, put in a large pan and cook with just the water clinging to the leaves for 4–5 minutes until wilted.

3. Transfer to a colander and drain thoroughly. When the spinach is cool enough to handle, gently squeeze out the excess liquid.

4. Put the pine nuts on a baking tray, and lightly toast under a medium grill for 2–3 minutes until golden brown – be careful not to scorch them.

5. Put the ricotta, spinach and eggs in a bowl, and mix together.

6. Add the pine nuts, beat well, then stir in the ground almonds and Parmesan.

7. Roll out the puff pastry into two squares, each about 8 in wide. Trim the edges, reserving the pastry trimmings.

8. Put one of the pastry squares on a baking tray. Spoon over the spinach mixture to within ½ in of the edge of the pastry.

9. Brush the edges with beaten egg, and put the second square over the top.
10. Using a round-bladed knife, press the pastry edges together by tapping along the sealed edge. Use the pastry trimmings to decorate the pie.
11. Bake in the oven for 10 minutes.
12. Reduce the oven temperature to 375°F, and bake for a further 25–30 minutes.
13. Serve hot.

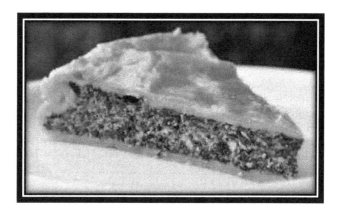

Vegetable Jalousie

Serves 4

Ingredients:

- 1,1 lb ready-prepared puff pastry
- 1 egg, beaten, to glaze

For the filling

- 1 oz butter
- 1 leek, finely chopped
- 2 garlic cloves, crushed
- 1 red pepper, seeded and sliced
- 1 yellow pepper, seeded and sliced
- 2 oz mushrooms, wiped with damp kitchen paper and sliced
- 3 oz small fresh asparagus spears, ends trimmed
- 2 tablespoons plain flour

- 3,5 fl oz vegetable stock
- 3,5 fl oz milk
- 4 tablespoons dry white wine
- 1 tablespoon chopped fresh oregano
- salt
- ground black pepper

Procedure:

1. Preheat the oven to 400°F.
2. Melt the butter in a frying pan, and sauté the leek and garlic, stirring frequently, for 2 minutes.
3. Add the peppers, mushrooms and asparagus, and cook for 3–4 minutes.
4. Add the flour and fry for 1 minute. Remove the pan from the heat, and stir in the vegetable stock, milk and white wine.
5. Return the pan to the heat and bring to the boil, stirring, until thickened. Stir in the oregano, and season with salt and pepper.
6. Roll out half of the pastry on a lightly floured surface to form a rectangle measuring 15 x 6in.

7. Roll out the other half of the pastry to the same shape, but a little larger all round. Put the smaller rectangle on a baking tray lined with dampened baking parchment.

8. Spoon the filling evenly on top of the smaller rectangle, leaving a 1/2 in margin around the edges.

9. Using a sharp knife, cut parallel diagonal slits across the larger rectangle to within 1 in on each of the long edges.

10. Brush the edges of the smaller rectangle with beaten egg, and place the larger rectangle on top, pressing the edges to seal.

11. Brush the whole jalousie with egg to glaze, and bake in the oven for 30–35 minutes until risen and golden.

12. Serve immediately.

Ratatouille

Ingredients:

- 2 large aubergines, coarsely chopped
- 4 courgettes, coarsely chopped
- 5 fl oz olive oil
- 2 onions, sliced
- 2 garlic cloves, chopped
- 1 large red pepper, seeded and coarsely chopped
- 2 large yellow peppers, seeded and coarsely chopped
- sprig of fresh rosemary
- sprig of fresh thyme
- 1 teaspoon coriander seeds, crushed
- 3 plum tomatoes, chopped
- 8 fresh basil leaves, torn
- salt
- freshly ground black pepper

Procedure:

1. Sprinkle the aubergines and courgettes with salt, then place them in a colander with a plate and a

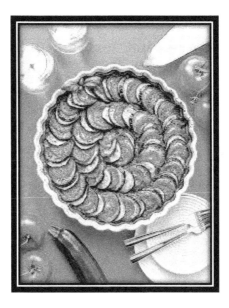

   weight on top to extract the bitter juices and excess water.

2. Leave to stand for about 30 minutes.

3. Heat the oil in a large heavy pan. Add the onions, sweat gently for 6–7 minutes until just softened, then add the garlic and sweat for another 2 minutes.

4. Rinse the aubergines and courgettes, and pat dry with kitchen paper.
5. Add to the pan with the peppers, increase the heat and sauté until the peppers are just turning brown.
6. Add the herbs and coriander seeds, then cover the pan and cook gently for about 40 minutes.
7. Add the tomatoes and season well with salt and pepper.
8. Cook gently for 10 minutes until the vegetables are soft but not too mushy.
9. Remove the herb sprigs. Stir in the basil leaves, and check the seasoning and serve hot.

Fusilli With Tomato & Mozzarella

Ingredients:

- 2,5 lb vine-ripened tomatoes, chopped
- 4 oz mozzarella cheese, diced
- 4 fl oz extra virgin olive oil
- 2 garlic cloves, chopped
- 20 large fresh basil leaves, torn into pieces
- 5 anchovy fillets in oil, drained and cut into small pieces
- 1/4 teaspoon chopped fresh oregano
- 1/2 teaspoon salt
- 1 lb dried fusilli
- freshly ground black pepper

Procedure:

1. Put the tomatoes in a serving bowl.
2. Add mozzarella, oil, garlic, basil, anchovies, oregano and salt. Season with pepper, and mix well.
3. Leave to marinate for 1–3 hours at room temperature to enable the flavours to mingle and develop.
4. Bring a large saucepan of salted water to the boil.
5. Cook the fusilli until al dente, stirring frequently to prevent sticking.
6. Drain and add to the bowl with the sauce, tossing everything together.
7. Serve immediately.

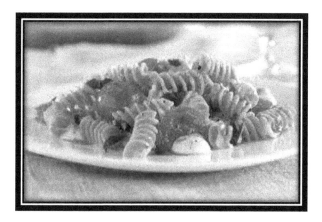

Sweet & Sour Tofu

Serves 4

Ingredients:

- 2 tablespoons vegetable oil
- 2 garlic cloves, crushed
- 2 celery sticks, sliced
- 1 carrot, cut into matchsticks
- 1 green pepper, seeded and diced
- 3 oz mangetout, halved
- 8 baby corn cobs
- 5 oz beansprouts
- 1 lb firm tofu, cubed

For the sauce

- 2 tablespoons soft brown sugar
- 2 tablespoons wine vinegar

105

- 8 fl oz vegetable stock
- 1 teaspoon tomato purée
- 1 tablespoon cornflour

Procedure:

1. Heat the vegetable oil in a preheated wok until it is almost smoking.
2. Reduce the heat slightly, then add the garlic, celery, carrot, pepper, mangetout and baby corn. Stir-fry for 3–4 minutes.
3. Add the beansprouts and tofu to the wok, and stir-fry for 2 minutes.
4. To make the sauce, combine the sugar, wine vinegar, stock, tomato purée and cornflour, stirring well to mix.
5. Stir into the wok, bring to the boil and cook, stirring, until the sauce thickens and turns glossy.
6. Continue for cook for 1 minute.
7. Serve immediately with rice or noodles.

Falafels

Ingredients:

- 1,75 lb canned cooked chickpeas, drained and rinsed
- 1/4 onion
- 2 garlic cloves
- 1/2 oz flat-leaf parsley leaves
- 1/2 oz fresh coriander leaves
- 1 teaspoon ground cumin
- 1 tablespoon freshly squeezed lemon juice
- 14 beaten egg
- about 2 tablespoons olive oil

For the dressing

- 1 small handful of fresh mint
- 1 garlic clove
- 7 oz Greek-style yogurt

- salt
- freshly ground black pepper

Procedure:

1. To make the falafels, purée the chickpeas, onion, garlic, parsley, coriander, cumin and lemon juice in a blender or food processor.

2. Turn the mixture into a bowl, and beat in the egg, then cover and chill in the refrigerator for 30–60 minutes, or longer if more convenient.

3. Preheat the oven to 350°F.

4. With wet hands, shape the mixture into 20 equal-size balls.

5. Put the falafels on an oiled baking sheet, and flatten them slightly, then brush with a little oil.

6. Bake in the oven for 20 minutes, turning the falafels over halfway through the cooking time.

7. To make the dressing, blend or process the mint, garlic and yogurt until smooth, turn into a bowl and season with salt and pepper.

8. To serve, put the falafels on a serving platter, and spoon the dressing over the top.

9. Serve hot.

Kidney Bean Kiev

Serves 4

Ingredients:

For the garlic butter

- 4 oz butter
- 3 garlic cloves, crushed
- 1 tablespoon chopped fresh flat-leaf parsley

For the bean patties

- 1,5 lb canned cooked red kidney beans, drained
- 5 oz fresh white breadcrumbs
- 1 oz butter
- 1 leek, chopped
- 1 celery stick, chopped
- 1 tablespoon chopped fresh flat-leaf parsley
- 1 egg, beaten
- vegetable oil for shallow-frying

- salt
- freshly ground black pepper

Procedure:

1. To make the garlic butter, put the butter, garlic and parsley in a bowl and blend together using a wooden spoon.
2. Put the garlic butter on a sheet of baking parchment, roll into a cigar shape and wrap in the baking parchment.
3. Chill in the refrigerator until required.
4. Using a potato masher, mash the red kidney beans in a mixing bowl and stir in half of the breadcrumbs until thoroughly blended.
5. Melt the butter in a heavy frying pan. Add the leek and celery, and sweat over a low heat, stirring constantly, for 3–4 minutes.
6. Add the bean mixture to the pan, together with the parsley and a pinch of salt. Mix thoroughly.
7. Remove the pan from the heat, and set aside to cool slightly.
8. Divide the kidney bean mixture into four equal portions, and shape them into ovals.

9. Slice the garlic butter into four pieces, and place a slice in the centre of each bean patty.
10. With your hands, mould the bean mixture around the garlic butter to encase it completely.
11. Dip each bean patty into the beaten egg to coat, then roll in the remaining breadcrumbs.
12. Heat a little oil in a frying pan over a medium heat, and fry the patties, turning once, for 7–10 minutes until golden brown.
13. Serve immediately.

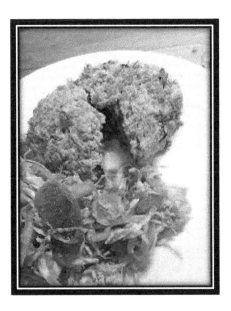

Veggie Burgers

Serves 2

Ingredients:

- 4 oz fresh green beans
- 4 oz bulgur wheatt
- 8 fl oz boiling water
- 1 small courgette
- 1 small carrot
- 1/2 Granny Smith apple
- 4 oz canned cooked chickpeas, rinsed and drained
- 1 tablespoon minced onion
- 1 tablespoon peanut butter
- 1,5 tablespoons vegetable oil
- 1/2 teaspoon curry powder
- 1/2 teaspoon chilli powder
- 4 oz fresh breadcrumbs

- salt
- freshly ground black pepper

Procedure:

1. Cook the green beans in boiling water until tender but still with a bite.
2. Refresh in cold water, drain and chop finely.
3. Cook the bulgur in boiling water for 1 minute. Remove from the heat, cover and leave to stand.
4. Grate the courgette and carrot, then peel, core and grate the apple.
5. Wrap in a clean tea towel and squeeze out excess moisture. Combine with the green beans in a mixing bowl.
6. In a blender or food processor, purée the chickpeas, onion, peanut butter, oil, curry powder and chilli powder until smooth. Season with salt and pepper. Add to the grated vegetables.
7. Drain the bulgur through a strainer, pressing with the back of a spoon to extract excess liquid. Add to the bowl.

8. Add the breadcrumbs and refrigerate for 1 hour.

9. With wet hands, shape the mixture into four burgers. Cook under a medium grill for 3 minutes on each side.

10. Serve hot.

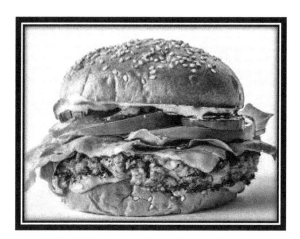

Tunisian Vegetables

Ingredients:

- 1 large aubergine, finely diced
- 4 tablespoons olive oil
- 1 large onion, finely chopped
- 2 garlic cloves, crushed
- 1 red pepper, seeded and diced
- 4 medium courgettes, diced
- 1 lb ripe tomatoes, chopped
- 2 tablespoons tomato purée
- 2 teaspoons chilli powder
- pinch of sugar
- salt
- freshly ground black pepper

Procedure:

1. Put the aubergine in a colander, sprinkle liberally with salt and cover with a plate or saucer.
2. Put a heavy weight on top, then leave for 30 minutes.
3. Rinse the aubergine under cold running water, then drain thoroughly.
4. Heat the oil in a large flameproof casserole dish, add the aubergine and onion, and cook gently, stirring frequently, until softened.
5. Add the garlic, pepper, courgettes and tomatoes. Stir well to mix, then pour in 10 fl oz water and bring to the boil, stirring.
6. Reduce the heat, then add the tomato purée, chilli powder and sugar. Season with salt and pepper.
7. Cover and simmer gently for 30 minutes, stirring occasionally and adding more water if the mixture becomes dry.
8. Taste and adjust the seasoning, before serving hot.

Spring vegetable stir-fry

Serves 4

Ingredients:

- 1 tablespoon groundnut oil
- 1 garlic clove, sliced
- 1 in piece of fresh root ginger, finely chopped
- 4 oz baby carrots
- 4 oz young fresh asparagus, cut into 3 in pieces
- 8 spring onions, trimmed and cut into 2 in pieces
- 4 oz cherry tomatoes
- 4 oz patty-pan squash, roughly chopped
- 4 oz baby corn
- 4 oz green beans, topped and tailed
- 4 oz sugarsnap peas, topped

For the dressing

- juice of 2 limes

- 1 tablespoon clear honey
- 1 tablespoon soy sauce
- 1 teaspoon sesame oil and tailed

Procedure:

1. Heat the groundnut oil in a wok or large heavy frying pan.
2. Add the garlic and ginger, and stir-fry for about 1 minute.
3. Add the carrots, patty-pan squash, baby corn and beans, and stir-fry for a further 3–4 minutes.
4. Next, add the peas, asparagus, spring onions and cherry tomatoes, and stir-fry for a further 1–2 minutes.
5. To make the dressing, mix all the ingredients together.
6. Add to the wok or pan, stir well, then cover the wok or pan.
7. Cook for 2–3 minutes more until the vegetables are tender but still crisp.
8. Serve immediately.

Vegetable paella

Ingredients:

- 2 small fennel bulbs, halved lengthways
- 8 oz cherry tomatoes, halved
- 3 tablespoons olive oil
- 2 teaspoons coriander seeds, crushed
- 1,5 pt vegetable stock
- 4 oz wild rice
- 7 oz long-grain white rice
- 2 tablespoons chopped fresh coriander leaves
- juice of 1/2 lemon
- salt
- freshly ground black pepper

Procedure:

1. Preheat the oven to 400°F.

2. Put the fennel and tomatoes in a roasting tin, drizzle with the oil and sprinkle with the coriander seeds. Season with salt and pepper.
3. Roast the vegetables, turning them once or twice, for 40 minutes or until tender.
4. Meanwhile, bring the stock to the boil in a large heavy saucepan.

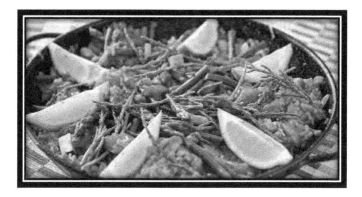

5. Add the wild rice and simmer for 30 minutes.
6. Add the long-grain rice and continue to cook for 15–20 minutes or until both types of rice are tender. Drain through a sieve.
7. Turn the rice and roasted vegetables into a large bowl, and toss to mix.
8. Sprinkle over the chopped coriander and lemon juice. Serve hot.

Courgette & asparagus parcels

Serves 4

Ingredients:

- 2 medium courgettes
- 1 medium leek
- 8 oz young fresh asparagus, trimmed
- 4 sprigs of fresh tarragon
- 4 whole garlic cloves, unpeeled
- 1 egg, beaten, to glaze
- salt
- freshly ground black pepper

Procedure:

1. Preheat the oven to 400°F.

2. Using a potato peeler, carefully slice the courgettes lengthways into thin strips.

3. Cut the leek into very fine julienne, and cut the asparagus evenly into 2 in lengths.

4. Cut out four sheets of baking parchment measuring 12 x 15 in and fold in half.

5. Draw a large curve to make a heart shape when unfolded. Cut along the line, and open out.

6. Divide the courgettes, asparagus and leek evenly between each paper heart, positioning the filling on one side of the fold line and topping each with a tarragon sprig and a garlic clove.

7. Season with salt and pepper.

8. Brush the edges lightly with the egg and fold over. Twist the edges together so that each parcel is completely sealed.

9. Lay the parcels on a baking tray, and cook in the oven for 10 minutes.

10. Serve immediately, laying the parcels on the serving plates to be opened at the table.

Leek & herb soufflé

Serves 4

Ingredients:

- 1 tablespoon olive oil
- 12 oz baby leeks, finely chopped
- 4 fl oz vegetable stock
- 2 oz walnuts
- 2 eggs, separated
- 2 tablespoons chopped fresh mixed herbs
- 2 tablespoons Greek-style yogurt
- salt
- freshly ground black pepper

Procedure:

1. Preheat the oven to 350°F. Lightly grease a 1,5 pt soufflé dish with vegetable oil.

2. Heat the olive oil in a frying pan. Add the leeks and sauté over a medium heat, stirring occasionally, for 2–3 minutes.

3. Add the stock to the pan, reduce the heat and simmer gently for a further 5 minutes.

4. Put the walnuts in a blender or food processor, and chop finely. Add the leek mixture to the nuts, and process briefly to form a purée. Transfer to a bowl.

5. Mix together the egg yolks, herbs and yogurt until thoroughly combined.

6. Pour the egg mixture into the leek purée. Season with salt and pepper, and mix well.

7. Put a baking tray into the oven to warm. In a separate bowl, whisk the egg whites until firm peaks form.

8. Gently fold the egg whites into the leek mixture. Spoon the mixture into the prepared dish, and place on the warmed baking tray.

9. Bake in the oven for 35–40 minutes until risen and set.

10. Serve immediately.

Broccoli with feta & tomato sauce

Ingredients:

- 1 lb broccoli, cut into florets
- 1 oz low-fat spread
- 1 large onion, finely chopped
- 3 garlic cloves, crushed
- 1,75 lb canned chopped plum tomatoes
- 1 teaspoon dried oregano
- 1 in piece of cinnamon stick
- 1 tablespoon freshly squeezed lemon juice
- 4 oz feta cheese, crumbled
- 4 oz Emmenthaler cheese, grated
- salt
- freshly ground black pepper

Procedure:

1. Preheat the oven to 375°F.
2. Cook the broccoli in lightly salted boiling water for 5 minutes until just tender.
3. Drain and place in an ovenproof serving dish.
4. Melt the low-fat spread in the saucepan. Sauté the onion and garlic for 3 minutes, stirring.
5. Add the tomatoes, oregano and cinnamon. Season with a little salt and pepper. Bring to the boil and simmer for 5 minutes. Discard the cinnamon stick.
6. Pour the sauce over the broccoli, and sprinkle with the lemon juice.
7. Sprinkle the two cheeses over the top.
8. Bake in the oven for 25 minutes, and serve.

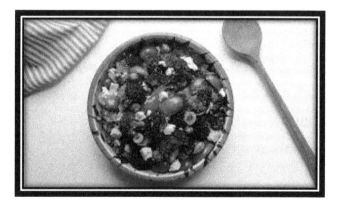

Chargrilled kebabs

Ingredients:

- 2 tablespoons freshly squeezed lemon juice
- 1 tablespoon olive oil
- 1 garlic clove, crushed
- 1 tablespoon chopped fresh rosemary leaves
- 1 red pepper, seeded and sliced into 1 in pieces
- 1 green pepper, seeded and sliced into 1 in pieces
- 1 yellow pepper, seeded andsliced into 1 in pieces
- 1 courgette, sliced into 1 in pieces
- 4 baby aubergines, quartered lengthways
- 2 red onions, each cut into 8 wedges
- salt
- freshly ground black pepper

Procedure:

1. If using bamboo skewers, soak in cold water for at least 30 minutes before using, to prevent them burning.

2. Put the peppers, courgette, aubergines and onions in a large bowl.

3. In another small bowl, whisk together the lemon juice, olive oil, garlic and rosemary.

4. Season with salt and pepper, and whisk again.

5. Pour the mixture over the vegetables, and stir to coat evenly.

6. Preheat the grill to medium. Thread the peppers, courgette, aubergines and onion alternately onto 8 skewers.

7. Arrange the kebabs on the grill rack, and cook for 10–12 minutes, turning frequently until the vegetables are lightly charred.

8. Serve hot.

Thank You!

Thank you so much for choosing my Ultimate Guide "Vegetarian Diet Recipes for Beginners", I've selected and cooked during my travels around the world!

To me these Vegetarian Recipes are absolutely the best, with the best flavors! And, of course, they are healthy dishes, so we can eat plenty of them.

I hope you enjoyed making the recipes as much as tasting them!

I'm already making a selection of the best Starters and Canapés for my next cookbook, so don't miss it!

CPSIA information can be obtained
at www.ICGtesting.com
Printed in the USA
BVHW081930250521
608097BV00001B/493